I0075801

What is Cancer?

by

Margaret M Stenerson

This book is dedicated to my

grandfather,

Harry Wold Stenerson,

a writer and a chemist.

INTRODUCTION

What a scary diagnosis! You may very well be terrified. You are looking for some answers. We will start with a simple question and go from there.

What is cancer? The simple answer is: a tumor, or a mass or a lesion. But where does it come from? To answer that question we have to look at your cells.

CHAPTER 1

Cell Structure

Cells are the building blocks of living things. All animals and plants have cells. A cell is the tiniest living unit.

For example, your skin has skin cells and nerve cells. You cannot see the cells in your skin without a microscope. If you have a microscope, even a child's microscope, you can probably see the cells in a piece of onion skin. The skin is the thin transparent layer between the onion parts.

Your blood has cells. You may have heard of red blood cells and white blood cells. They travel suspended in a clear liquid called plasma.

The Nucleus of a Cell

Every cell has a dark, dense, central core called the nucleus. Inside the nucleus is the material that determines your hair color and skin color and height. The DNA in the nucleus of a cell contains chromosomes that contain your genes. You get 23 chromosomes from your mother and 23 chromosomes from your father.

The DNA is **de**-oxy-ribo-**n**ucleic **a**cid. Each person has their own unique DNA. That is why they can use it during trials in court to identify someone.

Your DNA contains the instruction code for cells to divide. That is why your skin stays the same color. When you get new skin cells, they use the instructions in the DNA of your cells.

CHAPTER 2

What Causes Cancer?

Cancer is a disease characterized by out-of-control cell growth. Normal cells in the body follow an orderly path. They grow, they divide, and they die. Unlike normal cells, cancer cells do not experience programmed death. Instead, they continue to grow and divide.

Cells can experience uncontrolled growth if there are damages or mutations to the DNA. Therefore, there is damage to the genes that control cell division. There are four key genes responsible for the cell division process. They are:

- **Oncogenes** that tell the cells when to divide.

- **Tumor suppressor genes** that tell cells when not to divide.

- **Suicide genes** that control cell death. They tell the cell to kill itself if something goes wrong.

- **DNA-repair genes** that instruct a cell to repair damaged DNA.

Cancer occurs when a cell's gene mutations make the cell unable to correct DNA damage. The cell is unable to die. Cancer is also the result of mutations that inhibit the oncogenes' and tumor suppressor genes' to function. Thus, there is uncontrolled growth.

There are a variety of causes for cancer. They include:

- Carcinogens(cancer-causing substances)

- Age

- Genetic make-up

- The immune system

- Body weight

- Environment

- Viruses

- Bacteria

We will explain each one of these.

CHAPTER 3

Carcinogens

A carcinogen is a substance that can help cause cancer. Some known carcinogens are: tobacco and tobacco smoke, asbestos, and benzene, carbon tetrachloride and cadmium. For a complete list, go to this web site: http://www.cancer.org/docroot/PED/content/PED_1_3x_Known_and_Probable_Carcinogens.asp

Age

Most types of cancer become more common as we get older. This is because the changes that make a cell cancerous take a long time to develop. There has to be a number of changes to the genes in a cell before it turns into a cancer cell. The longer we live, the more time there is for mutations to occur.

Genetic Make-up

Sometimes a person is born with a genetic mutation. With one mutation, it is more likely that they will develop cancer during their lifetime. Doctors call this genetic predisposition.

The BRCA1 and BRCA2 breast cancer genes are examples of genetic predisposition. Women who carry one of these faulty genes have a greater chance of developing breast cancer than women who do not.

However, most breast cancer is not caused by a high-risk inherited gene fault. Researchers are looking at the genes of people with cancer. They hope to discover genes that are responsible for the cancer.

CHAPTER 4

Your Immune System

People who have trouble with their immune systems are more likely to get some type of cancer. This includes people who:

- Have had organ transplants and take drugs to suppress their immune systems.

- Have HIV or AIDS.

- Are born with rare medical syndromes that affect their immunity.

The types of cancer that affect these people include cervical cancer, lymphomas, liver cancer, and stomach cancer.

Body weight, Diet and Physical Activity

Cancer experts estimate that:

- Maintaining a healthy body weight

- Making changes to our diets

- Engaging in daily physical activity

could prevent one in three deaths from cancer.

Most people in the Western world eat too much red meat and processed meats. They do not eat enough fruits and vegetables. The Western type of diet seems to increase the risk of developing cancer.

CHAPTER 5

The Environment

Environmental causes of cancer include those substances around us every day. They include:

- Tobacco smoke
- The sun
- Natural and man-made radiation
- Work place hazards, such as chemicals
- Asbestos

Some of these you can avoid; others you cannot avoid. Most of them are only contributing factors. Scientists are trying to put the pieces of the puzzle together.

Viruses

Viruses seem to help to cause some cancers. But the cancer is not something you can "catch" from another person, such as a cold or flu virus. The virus can cause genetic mutations in your cells.

The following cancers and viruses are linked together.

- Cervical cancer and the genital wart virus – HPV (human papillomavirus)

- Primary liver cancer and the Hepatitis B and C viruses

- Lymphomas and the Epstein-Barr virus

- T-cell leukemia in adults and the Human T cell leukemia virus

- Oropharyngeal cancer and non-melanoma skin cancer and the HPV virus

Infection with any of these viruses increases the risk of getting cancer.

Scientists now believe that everyone with an invasive cervical cancer has had an HPV infection. Believe it or not, you could be infected with one of these cancer causing viruses, and never get cancer. That's the good news.

CHAPTER 6

Bacterial Infection

Bacterial infections are not thought of as cancer causing agents. Recent studies show that people with helicobacter pylori infection of their stomach develop inflammation of the stomach lining. This increases the risk of stomach cancer. Helicobacter pylori infection is usually treated with a combination of antibiotics.

Researchers are looking at whether substances produced by bacteria in the digestive system increase the risk of colon cancer. If bacteria prove to be cancer-causing agents, they can be treated with antibiotics. Cancer prevention would be possible.

CHAPTER 7

What Are the Symptoms of Cancer?

Cancer symptoms are very varied. They depend on where the cancer is.

- The symptom of breast cancer is any unusual lump in one of your breast.

- The symptom for colon cancer is probably blood in your stool.

- The symptom of skin cancer is an irregular mole.

- The symptom of prostate cancer is difficulty urinating.

- There are no symptoms for lung cancer.

Symptoms can be created as the tumor grows and pushes against other organs and blood vessels. As cancer cells use the body's energy, they can interfere with normal functioning.

It is possible to present the following symptoms.

- Fever

- Fatigue

- Excessive sweating

- Anemia

- Unexplained weight loss

When the cancer spreads, it metastasizes, that means it spreads to other parts of the body. Additional symptoms can be present. Swollen or enlarged lymph nodes are common. If cancer spreads to the brain, you may experience:

- Vertigo (dizziness)

- Headaches

- Seizures

Cancer spreading to the lungs may cause hoarseness and shortness of breath. The liver may become enlarged and cause jaundice (yellow skin and eyes). Bones can become painful, brittle and break easily. Symptoms, again, depend on the location in your body.

CHAPTER 8

Malignancies

Malignancies are cancerous tumors. A benign tumor is non-cancerous. The only way your doctor can know if there is a malignancy is by doing a biopsy of the tumor. This involves taking a small piece of the tumor from the body. Usually it is done with a needle.

Then, a pathologist, who is an expert in cell identification, looks at your cells using a microscope. The cells will either be normal or cancerous. That is the only way to identify a malignancy.

Even a mammogram, which may find a small lesion in one of your breasts, or micro-crystallization will need to be biopsied.

Malignant tumors form in either of two ways.

1. A cancerous cell manages to move throughout the body in the blood or lymph system. It

destroys healthy tissue during this invasion.

2. A cancer manages to divide and grow. It makes new blood vessels to feed itself. This process is angiogenesis.

Once metastasis develops, the cancer is very hard to treat. Treatment types for cancer are covered in other e-books for sale on Kindle.

CHAPTER 9

Conclusion

We have answered the question, "What is cancer?" by teaching you a little about cells in your body. We discussed the variety of causes for cancer and the symptoms of cancer.

Malignancies need treatment. You may want to buy one of our other e-books for more specific information.

My other e-books are listed here. They are chock full of facts in an easy to read style. No fancy medical terms are used. You would find these books exceptionally helpful for you and your family.

The price is reasonable and you can have your purchase right away. Just a few keystrokes and it is yours for the asking.

Amazon KDP Books

Complementary and Alternative Medicine for Lung Cancer

A Cancer Patient's Guide to Hospitals

Colonoscopy Preparation

Nutrition and Cancer

Breast Cancer Diet

A Cancer Patient's Guide to Decision Making and End-of-Life Issues

CHAPTER 10

Complementary and Alternative Medicine for Lung Cancer

If you are diagnosed with cancer and you are wondering what else is out there to help me, this e-book may be for you. It describes in detail some non-traditional ways to deal with your cancer.

The book starts with some facts and information about complementary therapies, and then, about alternative therapies.

Chapter 2 is all about a historical look at some of the therapies that people have used.

Chapter 3 describes each of nine complementary therapies used along side conventional treatments. These therapies will help you cope with the disease and bring you some peace of mind.

Chapter 4 is a discussion of Indian medicine, Ayurvedic medicine. It is an interesting alternative to conventional therapy. There are two other alternative therapies described in detail.

Chapter 5 is specific for your type of cancer. It covers:

- Breast cancer
- Colon cancer
- Lung Cancer
- Prostate cancer
- Skin cancer

You would buy the book that is appropriate for your type of cancer.

Each type of cancer has specific remedies that may or may not help you. We explain them in detail.

This is an interesting e-book to have. It informs you of all the possible alternatives to standard treatments. You want to gain as much information as you can so you can make intelligent decisions. You will not find all this information in any one place on the Web. Buy this book. You won't be disappointed. Learn to help yourself!

CHAPTER 11

A Cancer Patient's Guide to Hospitals

This e-book is a must read for cancer patients. It is such a valuable tool. It is not just about hospitals. It covers health insurance plans and ratings for doctors.

Chapter 1 explains the different health insurance plans. It helps you figure out what the insurance will pay for.

Chapter 2 is all about rating your doctor. You will find out how to check on a doctor's credentials and his rating as well.

Chapters 3 through 6 deal with hospital ratings, mortality rates, and specialties. It helps you decide if you want to go to a teaching hospital. There are links to web sites to help you learn about your hospital.

Chapter 7 and 8 explain travel and accommodations at hospitals. It discusses the four Cancer Treatment Centers of America that are seen in advertisements on television.

Finally, there is a report card of sorts to help you assign a grade to your hospital. In the Appendix of the book is information about the major cancer centers in the United States.

The major cancer centers are located in New York City, Boston, Los Angeles,

San Francisco, Seattle and Houston. Each one of them is discussed in detail.

You cannot afford to be without this e-book. It will guide you as you choose where to have your cancer treatment. There are so many factors to consider.

All of this varied information is in one place for you. You could not go to any one web site and accumulate this knowledge.

I offer a money-back guarantee. You have nothing to lose. You will not be disappointed.

CHAPTER 12

Colonoscopy Preparation

Here is an e-book for everybody over the age of 50. Colonoscopies are recommended once every ten years at a minimum. A colonoscopy is not just for people who might have cancer. It is for everybody.

The book opens with a brief history of colonoscopies. There is a chapter about your digestive system in general. Then there is a chapter about your colon. It explains where it is and how it works.

The e-book describes a colonoscopy preparation diet. It contains suggestions to get you ready for the exam. We give you a little bit more information than your doctor's instructions.

Chapter 5 is all about bowel disorders. You will read about polyps in your colon and the different types of polyps. You will also learn about diverticulitis.

There is a chapter that addresses the safety of colonoscopies. You will find out how to locate a center near you.

Finally there are many recipes you can use to increase the amount of fiber you eat. They are nutritious and easy to follow.

All in all, this is a wonderful e-book that prepares you for your colonoscopy. The more you know, the less fearful you will be.

Be kind to yourself and purchase this e-book for your peace of mind. I offer a money-back guarantee. You have nothing to lose. I predict you will not be disappointed.

CHAPTER 13

Nutrition and Cancer

The title of this e-book does not do justice to all the information it contains. There is so much to learn. What does cancer do to my digestion of food? What is the best way to deal with side effects?

Chapter 1 is an introduction to nutrition in general. What nutrients are necessary to deal with this disease?

There are lists of suggestions for you to try. Guidelines help you prepare for meals after surgery or treatment.

Chapter 2 is all about the effects of cancer. How does surgery affect you? How will chemotherapy affect you? What about radiation? What can you do to alleviate the discomfort of advanced cancer?

Chapter 3 is all about symptom relief. It describes the best way to deal with side effects of treatment. The e-book describes the best way to deal with mouth sores, diarrhea, and poor appetite. There are others explained here also.

Chapter 4 has some pro-active steps you can take to lower your risk of cancer. There are specific suggestions for different types of cancer. You can read about your particular disease.

Finally, there are recipes to help you cope with your cancer. Then, there are lists to help you know what foods are beneficial and what foods you should avoid. There are suggestions for supplements you can take that may be helpful.

This e-book will become your guide to healthy eating. You will find the information very valuable.

We offer you a money-back guarantee. You have nothing to lose by buying this e-book.

Help yourself to feel better and get the nutrition you need.

CHAPTER 14

A Cancer Patient's Guide to Decision-Making and End-of-Life Issues

This e-book is not necessarily for cancer patients only. It is a guide that everyone can use. The information is not limited in its application.

This Guide will show you how to:

- Prepare a Health Care Proxy

- Make out a Living Will or a Medical Power of Attorney

- Gather documents

- Make out a Last Will and Testament

- Assign a Power of Attorney

- Establish a Living Trust

- Avoid Taxes

- Find a Lawyer

- Consider Social Security

- Plan for your funeral

At the end of each chapter are links to web sites that you may find helpful.

We give you prices for some web documents you may want to use.

What is the difference between a living will and a regular will? All of these things are explained in detail.

If you are a spouse or sibling of someone with cancer, you will find this information invaluable. The cancer patient himself may not be able to deal with these issues directly. You may be able to help him.

This e-book will not disappoint you either. You will be happy with your purchase. And, you will share the information with family members. This is an investment for your children and grandchildren.

The **website address for the e-books is:**

http://www.amazon.com/kdp/books

If you do not have access to a computer, the public library is a choice. Or you can ask a neighbor, or a son, or daughter, or grandchildren to get the KDP e-books for you. Once they are

downloaded to a computer then you
can print them.

Please e-mail me if you have any
questions:

stenersonmargaret@yahoo.com

www.ingramcontent.com/pod-product-compliance
Lightning Source LLC
Chambersburg PA
CBHW032019190326
41520CB00007B/535